<u>4thgc.com</u> - presents
(OFFICIAL TRAINING GUIDE)
Online Marketing
FOR HOME HEALTH CARE

authored by
Tim Beachum & Chris Beachum

Copyright 2014 Tim Beachum | 4th Generation Communications
Copyright Notice

© Copyright 4th Generation Communications LLC. 2014

ALL RIGHTS RESERVED.
No part of this report can be reproduced or distributed in any way without written permission of the author.

DISCLAIMER AND/OR LEGAL NOTICES:
The information presented herein represents the view of the author as of the date of publication. Because of the rate with which conditions change, the author reserves the right to alter and update his opinion based on the new conditions. The report is for informational purposes only.

While every attempt has been made to verify the information provided in this report, neither the author nor his affiliates/partners assume any responsibility for errors, inaccuracies or omissions.

Any slights of people or organizations are unintentional. If advice concerning legal or related matters is needed, the services of a fully qualified professional should be sought. This report is not intended for use as a source of legal or accounting advice.

You should be aware of any laws which govern business transactions or other business practices in your country and state. Any reference to any person or business whether living or dead is purely coincidental.

CONSUMER NOTICE: You should assume that the author of this report has an affiliate relationship and/or another material connection to the providers of goods and services mentioned in this report and may be compensated when you purchase from a provider. You should always perform due diligence before buying goods or services from anyone via the Internet or offline.

Our Definition of Marketing

Here's the traditional definition of marketing:

mar·ket·ing
/märkədiNG/

noun

the action or business of promoting and selling products and selling products or services, including market research and advertising.

Here is my definition:

Using a clear cut strategy to help a company to gain more targeted exposure. The more exposure a name brand receives, the more of authority it will become in their particular niche.

Increased targeted exposure online, will lead to more targeted traffic, which leads to more leads, which leads to more sales.

Free 30-Minute Consultation

Once you have finished reading this guide you are entitled to a free consultation. I do not want this guide to be just another book in your collection of useless books. I want you to actually make money.

In order to make sure that you are successful, I want to give you a free 30-minute consultation via telephone. I want to make sure that no rock has been left unturned. You will have no excuse for not succeeding.

In order to claim your free consultation go to the following URL and fill out the form. I will personally contact you to set up a mutual time.

Free 30-Minute Consultation claim form:

http://www.4thgc.com/consultation

Introduction

I know you are excited and ready to dive right in. I have had the privilege of speaking with home health care providers for more than a decade. In fact my mother is one of them. She has had me volunteering in the field every since I was a kid.

My mother is still in the business, as a nurse and a consultant. It still amazes me how many doctors call her for advice. It also amazes me that I am a grown man and she still volunteers my services. I respectfully remind her that I am grown and that I am now paid at least $500 an hour for my consulting services.

Guess what???

I still speak to many medical facilities and help them get on track with their marketing absolutely free — all because momma told me to do it. :-)

This marketing guide was created to help business owners in the health care industry. It doesn't matter if you own a private pay facility with one client, or you have dreams of expanding, or you already own and operate a multi-patient facility. This guide will help you to increase your health care business's exposure.

My promise to you

There are a ton of marketing books on the market. The problem with most of them is this — they are based on theory, or outdated materials.

I promise you that the information in this guide **will** increase your websites online visibility. I will give you a clear cut blueprint to help you jump start your home health care business.

The information within the pages of this guide is based on a training workshop that my son and I have performed for business owners from around the world. We have always talked about creating a book and sharing it with other business owners, but like most things in life it was one of those things we kept saying we would start tomorrow - and as you know tomorrow never came.

It wasn't until my son mentioned that he was sick and tired of hearing all of the horror stories about home health care professionals that were taken advantage of by scrupulous marketers. These snakes were making their living by lying to hard working people just like you.

We realized that there were only so many workshops that we can do in a year. There was no way that we could reach every single home health care agency that needed us. We decided to take our workshop and pour it into this training guide. We also made it extremely easy to understand. .

As a home health care professional you have taken an oath to save, and improve the quality of peoples lives. You do not have the time to study all of the changes that happens online on a daily basis.

Chances are you have put your faith in other marketers and ended up disappointed. By the time you have finished reading this guide you will have the knowledge necessary to qualify a good marketing company. You will even have the ability to train a staff member to effectively do the job. You will know what questions to ask, you will be well versed in marketing industry lingo. In a nutshell you will be able to weed through any over hyped sales information that will be thrown your way.

It is important for me to tell you right up front, that this guide isn't for someone who just wants to do good in their market. It is designed to help you totally annihilate your niche market.

You want to become the brand in your market space that everyone comes to. If you are not willing to walk the cutting edge and totally dominate your market, then this guide is not for you.

How To Use This Guide

You are holding in your hands over a decade of experience. I have had the privilege of speaking with individuals in the home health care industry from around the world. After 10+ years of training, consulting and doing workshops, it is safe to say that I have discovered a few patterns that those in the home health care industry have in common when it comes to marketing their businesses online.

The number one pattern that I have seen in the home health among business owners is that they are way to busy running their businesses, and do not have time to keep up with the rapid changes going on in their industry online. I wrote this guide to level the playing field for you.

Even if you do not plan on marketing your business yourself, this guide will at least give you the knowledge to hire the right marketing company.

This guide contains the same strategies that I use for my personal online businesses, as well as my clients.

It is crucial to the future of your business that you put aside what you think you may know about marketing. I want you to approach this guide with a clean slate. Chances are some of the strategies that I am going to share with you will go against everything that the majority of marketing "*experts*" are preaching.

I highly recommend that you read this guide cover to cover (*even if you are not planning to manage your own online presence*). If there is a term that you do not understand, check the glossary in the back of the guide.

Keep in mind that this is not a "*how to*" guide. It is meant to help you either improve your current marketing efforts, or implement some new strategies to help you generate more leads.
Once you have completed reading this guide - then and only then should you dive in and start implementing the

strategies. It is important that you understand the big picture.

In the next section entitled, "*Why Internet Marketing Is Crucial For The Home Health Care Industry*". I want to make a few things clear. I want to make sure that we are on the same page. This is a crucial chapter and is considered the foundation of everything else that will be covered later on in this guide.

I also want you to know that I am here if you need me. You can simply call my business line. If I am unable to answer leave a message and I will return your call as soon as possible.

Here is my number: 757-271-5605

Why Internet Marketing Is Crucial For The Home Health Care Industry

I have spoken to business owners from all sizes and walks of life. I am talking about business owners who make custom wedding tuxedos for small and miniature dogs, to hair restoration specialists looking to become an authority in their niche. When I ask them why is Internet Marketing important to their business, I am told, "*Internet Marketing is important because it increases the company's profits.*"

The funny thing is most business owners believe that the only purpose that marketing serves is to generate a profit for their business. If you are one of those business owners who share this belief thats fine — its not your fault. You, like other business owners across the world have been mislead. Your profit is generated from the products and or services that you sale.

The purpose of marketing is to give your brand exposure. To be more specific, marketing done right will give your brand exposure in front of your target audience.

At first glance it may appear that I said the same thing twice. The key phrase here is "target audience". It does not matter how much exposure your business receives, if it is in front of the wrong people.

The primary focus of your Internet Marketing should be first and foremost, building your brand. When I say that to most business owners they have a look of shock on their face. Building your brand will ensure long term profits, as well as stability in your market place.

Allow me to prove myself. Have you ever heard the name Ralph Lifshitz? Most people do not recognize the name. He is a business owner who didn't think his name had enough marketability, so he changed it to Ralph Lauren. Does that name ring a bell now? He is the owner and founder of the Polo brand. There are a variety of clothing brands on the market, with new brands popping up daily. However, Polo is a brand recognized world wide.

15 minutes can save you 15% or more on car insurance. What's the name of the company with that slogan? Its obviously Geico. This car insurance company figured out a way to grab your attention long enough to sale you car insurance. They are one of the most popular car insurance companies in America. Why? Because of their name branding efforts.

I was at the gym a few days ago, and right next to me were two guys debating about smartphones. The one guy said that his Galaxy Samsung was the best smartphone on the market. The other guy proudly stated that he was and always will be an Apple man. He went on to boast about all of the Apple products he had. This does nothing but prove that Apple is hands down the quintessential example of what brands should strive to be like.

Do you understand the importance of building your brand? Are you starting to see the power of name branding done right? You can easily start building your name brand by adding your logo and slogan to your site. It should be the first thing that people see when they hit your website. It should also be on every page of your site.

Take a few minutes to research your competitors websites. You are going to be blown away by how many of your competitors are doing nothing to build their name brand. This is something that you can easily apply to your internet marketing to give you that cutting edge over and above the competition.

If you are already using traditional forms of advertising such as television, radio, and print that is a good start. Although traditional advertising isn't what it use to be it still serves a purpose. In order to be successful you have to be everywhere your prospective customers are. The reality of marketing is your customers are turning away from television, radio, and print media, because they can find everything they want on the internet. As I mentioned just a moment ago, traditional marketing still has its uses. It is however, important for you to be prepared for the digital transition. If you have Hulu then you have seen the commercials that come on during your show. That my friend is the future of television.

The majority of magazines and news papers that you enjoy — if not already will soon be in digital format. As you sit there reading this guide, traditional advertising is making the transition to the digital world. Like it or not it is the direction your prospects are moving. It is crucial that you are there to greet them.

Consumers making online purchases or researching the best service in their local area has increased over the last few years. Lets face it, we all live extremely busy lifestyles, and convenience is a top priority. Most people do not have time to call around to see who offers the best service or who has the lowest price. People today do not care to drive around from place to place looking to see who has a particular name brand item on sale. It's way easier to "*Google it*".

Internet marketing is one of the most cost-effective methods of marketing as compared to traditional forms of marketing. Just like any other form of marketing its all about having consistent exposure in your market place.

Internet marketing allows you to have a 24/hour sales person working for you. Your digital sales rep will deliver information about your products and or services at the convenience of your prospect.

If done right internet marketing casts a wide net online. It allows you to show up in search results for a variety of search terms. If your prospect is sitting in the waiting room waiting on his or her doctors appointment they should be able to easily research your product/services. If your prospect has problems sleeping at 4am in the morning, he or she should be able to find the desired information they are looking for regarding your business and what you have to offer.

With other forms of advertising you can not change directions on a whim. With traditional forms of marketing once your offer is out in the world its out there. You would have to redo your ad and launch another marketing campaign which will cost you a lot of money. However with Internet marketing you can easily logon to your website and make changes and update it within minutes.

Internet marketing if done correctly gives you a massive amount of exposure. The more exposure you receive the more traffic you receive to your website. Each page on your website becomes a digital sales person. The content on each page gives you a chance to educate the consumer. The more you educate the consumer on what it is you have to offer the more you increase the odds of the consumer doing business with you.

It is a fact that consumers will use several different search terms when looking for information on a particular product or service.

Here is a real life example taken from one of our case studies. It is a prospect who is searching for a carpet cleaning service in their local area. Here is how they performed their searches:

- **First Search** - best carpet cleaning service
- **Second Search** - best carpet cleaning service for pet odor
- **Third Search** - best carpet cleaning service for pet stains
- **Fourth Search** - best carpet cleaning service for pet urine

Most people begin their searches by performing a general search. As they continue researching, their search will become more specific. Do you see the benefits of showing up for all four search terms in the example above?

Marketing is all about getting the most exposure possible. This is a phrase that you will hear me repeating over and over again throughout this guide.

Are you starting to see why Internet Marketing is crucial to your business?

A Step-by-Step Blueprint

For this section you are going to need to take a few notes. You are also going to need some sort of idea of how your site is doing before you begin applying the strategies that I am about to share with you.

With that said and done — lets dive right in.

Name Branding

Most small business owners are so focused on getting their business up and running that name branding usually isn't at the top of their to-do list.

Every company needs a logo and a slogan. This allows your prospects to quickly identify your company. With constant exposure and a little creativity, prospects will associate your logo and slogan with your business over time.

You should have both your logo and slogan on every page of your site. The most effective location is the top left corner of your site, on all the pages.

This is the first thing that the visitor sees when they visit your site.

Lead Generator

You should have your lead form on every page of your site. The form needs to be located somewhere towards the top fold of the page. It should be clear that the form is for a free consultation, free estimate or whatever it is that you are offering. This is known as a lead funnel or a hook. (*Because the forms offer is used to hook the prospect.*)

There are however, exceptions to this rule. We have accomplished amazing results by adding a lead form at the end of the sites articles along with a call to action e.g. complete the form below to receive exclusive discount offers, for a free no hassle consultation etc. I think you get the point.

Keyword Research

Most business owners or marketing companies will blindly generate content for their site. Content that will never be seen by anyone. This is a huge waste of time. You should never create any content without first doing keyword research.

By doing keyword research you will know exactly what and how your prospects are performing searches for your products and or services. Once you have compiled a list of targeted keyword phrases, then and only then is it time to start creating content.

Do a search for some of the keyword phrases that you have discovered. Make a list of the competitors that you find in the top search results. Later on I will show you how to spy on them and what you will need to do to take their positions.

Content Schedule

You should have a monthly content schedule for developing and posting content. Each page on your website is like a billboard for your business. The more billboards you have strategically placed the more traffic you will generate, and the more leads and sales you will receive.

When referring to content I am talking about articles, social media posts, and videos. All of the above are the types of content that you should be creating to help push your site.

I will give you more information on the best practices for each content method a little later in this guide. For now I want you to remember that consistency is the key. Let me give you a quick simplified understanding of how search engines index your site.

Search engines have what is known as bots or spiders that constantly search the internet looking for new content to add to their search results. When they come to your site they follow all of the links to determine how many pages you have. Whenever the bots return they will see if any new content was added to your site. If your site is not updated on a regular basis the bots will slow down the rate in which they visit your site.

So, what does this mean?

If you only post fresh optimized content every other month, the spiders may only return to index those new pages two or three times a year if that. The more content you generate, the more the search engines will return to your site, the more pages you will get indexed, the more exposure your business will receive, which increase the odds of more visitors to your site.

Lets Focus On Google

The facts are the facts — Google is the largest search engine on the face of the planet. Without doing anything the rest of the search engines will follow suit and index your pages. The amount of time that this takes may vary.

Now that you understand the important roll that Google plays in the success of your site, lets see how your site is currently looking in Google's index.

Go to Google right now, and enter the following:

site:yourdomain.com

Make sure that you type everything altogether with no spaces. Where it says, "*yourdomain.com*" you enter your website's URL. Once you click the search button you will see the word "*About*" underneath the search box, along with a number. The number that you see under the search box is an approximation of how many pages your site has indexed in Google currently.

Ask yourself this..

Are you happy with the number of webpages you currently have indexed in Google?

Most local business owners have less than 300 pages indexed in Google, and they wonder why their business isn't doing so well.

As more websites begin competing for your search terms, the harder it will be for you to dominate the search engines.

Take a second to write down how many pages Google currently has indexed for your website. It is important to note that this number changes constantly. In the past I have seen it change two or three times a day.

Spying On The Competition

Make a list of your top competitors based on the keyword phrase you want to target. You will also want to note how many pages your competitors have indexed in Google currently. You will also want to note the content on their websites. Complete the competition spy list below:

1. How many of your competitors have a logo and a slogan prominently placed on each of their pages - above the fold?

2. How many of your competitors have a phone number displayed at the top of every page?

3. How many of your competitors have Google maps on their site? **TIP: Google tends to favor sites using their tools. Go figure!**

4. How many pages do your competitors have indexed? This

gives you an idea of how many targeted pages you will have to create in order to take them out.

5. Is the content educational? Business owners tend to use terms that are over the reader's head, or industry specific (*more on how your content should be written later*).

6. Note the keyword phrases that your competitors are using. Make sure to add them to your keyword list if you do not already have them on your list.

7. Rate your competitors navigation on a scale of 1 to 10. Is it easy to find your way around on their site or do you find it to be difficult?

(*You can download our free competitors spy list here: http://www.4thgc.com/mflbo/*)

Do not just skip over this part, it is crucial that you complete this exercise. By finding the answers to the above questions it will give you a birds-eye view of what your market looks like. It will let you know exactly what it is that you need to do in order to take over your local market. It will also allow you to see your progression over time.

I am always asked by clients and prospects, how long will it take before you start seeing results. There is no way that any marketer on the face of the planet can answer this question with any level of accuracy. You would have to have the ability to control several factors e.g. the search engines, how soon your backlinks are indexed, the actions of your website visitors etc.

What I can guarantee you is that once you get the strategies in this guide down to a science you will increase the exposure of your business.

Chances are you have spoken to a lot of marketers, and the majority of them probably tried to make marketing sound like a difficult process. Well the truth is it's not difficult, it is however systematic.

Ok it's time to back track and go into a little more detail about some of the things that I mentioned above. Let's start with your website.

Your Website's Foundation

NOTE: *The following information is advice based on my personal experience. I have achieved great success not only for my personal businesses but for clients from around the world using the exact same strategies that I am about to share with you.*

There are many ways you can build a website, but we recommend that our clients use Wordpress. My entire internet empire is built on Wordpress, and we have been using it for years. I highly recommend that if you are not using Wordpress that you consider switching to it. Wordpress is a free CMS (*content management system*) that is used worldwide. In fact, the large majority of websites online are built using the Wordpress platform.

From this point on I am going to assume that you are either using the Wordpress platform, or you plan on using it in the near future.

As you grow your business, and you start to gain more popularity in the search engines, there will be hackers and spammers waiting to take advantage of your site's success. Once you install Wordpress it comes with *Akismet,* which is a plugin that helps to protect your blog from comment and trackback spam automatically.

NOTE: *Just like any security program Akismet is not 100% guaranteed against spam attacks. It will however aid in reducing the amount of spam that you would normally get.*

Google Analytics - this is another software that allows you to track your website traffic, and a ton of other statistics. You can sign up for a free Google account if you do not already have one. If you currently have any type of Google account as of the writing of this book you will have access to all of Google's tools.

Once you have signed up for an account, you can download the Google Analytics plugin (*perform a web search for the Google Analytics plugin*).

Contact Form 7 - you will use this Wordpress plugin to build your forms. This is the form plugin we use to build your lead funnels.

Yet Another Related Posts Plugin - Adds related posts to your site and RSS feeds. This is an easy way to link your pages together, and it also helps the user find other related content. Another hidden secret of this little gem is that it helps improve the overall rankings of your website's pages.

WP Legal Pages - This is a 1 click legal page management plugin. It allows you to quickly add legal pages to your Wordpress sites.

The disclaimer is something that is often forgotten while building a website. WP Legal Pages is a basic disclaimer and will cover your butt if the stuff hits the fan. Its better to have it and not need it, rather than need it and not have it.

WordPres SEO - This is a quick little plugin that makes it brain-dead simple for you to optimize your content. Simply follow the instructions that come with the plugin.

StatPress - This offers realtime stats for your website. You will have the ability to see when the search engine spiders visit, and when people come to your site from the search engines.

The cool thing about Wordpress is that it can be customized a million different ways. The plugins that I recommended above is what I use on a daily basis. However there are thousands of plugins that you can use. Chances are, if you can dream up something that you want your website to do, or a feature that you wish you had, you will be able to find a plugin that can do it for you.

TIP: *There are plenty of videos on YouTube that will show you how to find and install plugins for Wordpress.*

Choosing The Right Theme

When it comes to Hair Loss Specialists, looks are everything. The same principal applies to your website. You do not get a second chance to make a good impression. This is another reason why I highly recommend using WordPress as your content management platform.

Wordpress has what is known as themes. The themes module controls the look and feel of your website. The good news is there are thousands of themes that are 100% free for you to choose from. However, it is important to note that free means that other people are also using the theme. The odds of your competitors using the same theme are pretty good.

Here are a couple of resources where you can check out some free themes:

- http://www.wpexplorer.com/top-free-themes/

- http://theme.wordpress.com/themes/sort/free/

- http://www.wpulti.net/best-free-wordpress-themes/

- http://colorlib.com/wp/free-wordpress-themes/

That should be enough to get you started. I highly recommend that you choose what is known as a responsive theme. A responsive them automatically adjust for mobile devices.

Currently 60% of Americans use a mobile device to access the internet. This number is growing by leaps and bounds every year. This is also traffic that you as a business owner do not want to miss out on.

Ideas For Creating Great Content

As far as generating visitors to your site, content is hands down the king. The days of being able to generate a bunch of garbage and getting it to rank is over. The days of creating content simply to bait the search engine spiders are also over. Producing educational, and enticing content that engages your visitors, is the brand-new model and personally should have been the business model from the very beginning. High quality, targeted content is an excellent method to build brand-awareness and its good for search engine optimization. As I pointed out earlier you should have a content schedule in place.

Companies that produce content on a consistent basis receive 55% more website site visitors and 97% more inbound links to their website than websites that do not. If you take a second to think about it - it all makes sense. If somebody finds the content on your website useful, they are more probable to have a look at your site for more information. They are also more likely to share your site with others.

Not Sure Exactly What Type Of Content To Develop?

One of the major difficulties facing business owners is how to create content that is interesting to their visitors and provide it in a manner that is entertaining and pertinent.

More often than not we hear business owners asking the question, "*where do I discover content to write about to keep the site visitors coming?*"

Fear no more! I will show you our "*7 No-brainer Content Developing Strategies*" to help you develop magnetic content on demand.

1. **Write about your products and or services**

Your products and or services are the focus of your company so this is an excellent chance to talk about what makes you different than your competitors. It is important to note, that when you are writing about your products or services you should avoid being self-promoting. Your prospects do not know you and do not want to be sold to. They are simply looking for information.

Content Ideas:

- You can write about an upcoming product launch. People love to be the first to know about something new. (*This can also be a service.*)

- Create infographics explaining the benefits of your products and or services.

2. Your opinions do not matter, its all about the client

Something that companies commonly ignore are their clients. As business owners, we often get caught up in the day-to-day cycle of our businesses. Because we are so busy, we often forget about grooming our prospects. You can easily leverage the power of your site by informing your customers about how your products and or services will help them. Without prospects you do not have clients. It would best serve you to ask your clients what is it that "they" want.

Content Ideas:

- Use your site to address concerns you get from consumers.
- Run a poll on a subject and write a post about the result.

- Are you thinking about introducing a new product? How about asking for feedback from your clients and prospects.

Take for example, a San Francisco-based clothing company, ModCloth. They opened up their website, and allowed their clients to vote on the items that their business should carry. ModCloth has actually taken the concept of co-creation to a brand-new level by creating a whole collection of user-generated designs. How's that for thinking out of the box?

3. Join the discussion on LinkedIn.

LinkedIn Groups are a fantastic place to discover and participate in discussions that can give you ideas for great content for your website. Just like forums, similar business experts are continuously linking and asking concerns in the '*Answers*' section of LinkedIn.

4. Write about industry-related trends and developments

You need to currently have a twitter account, if not, go sign up for one now. Once you have your Twitter account it is time to find a few leaders in your industry and follow them. Do the same for some of your major competitors. If you have a specialty piece of equipment make certain to follow the company that developed it on Twitter. If there are magazines that specializes in your niche, make sure to follow them as well.

NOTE: You need to do more than just follow users on Twitter, you must turn on your notifications. This will certainly allow you to be updated whenever the user post something to their timeline.

I know the media, as well as the majority of high profile marketers are screaming Facebook, but trust me when I say Twitter is the best tool for following trends and developments in your industry.

Proof of Twitters power - When Michael Jackson was rushed to the hospital, Twitter is how the world heard about it first. When Robbin Williams committed suicide, Twitter is how the world knew about it first. When Joan Rivers passed away, do you know where it broke first? Yep, Twitter! If it's breaking news in your industry, or new development chances are it will break on Twitter first.

5. **Read related industry blogs**

Read other niche related websites. Study the quality of content on their website, and take note of what you feel will appeal to your readers. Create similar content for your website. Research what they are doing, and create concepts for your own site (*do not EVER copy someones content verbatim*).

Another great technique to discover websites associated with your business is to browse Google for a keyword phrase specific to your niche market, and include the "*blog site*" to the end of your search.

Example: keyword phrase "*blog site*"

Content Ideas:

- Write about a current news item in your industry that brings about changes.
- Write about trends that may affect your industry or clients.
- Review a recently-published book from your industry.
- List and review applications or sites useful to your industry.

6. Turn your clients into celebrities

Why are your clients using your products and or services? Does it make them feel better, or look better? This is an opportunity to highlight your clients and make them celebrities for your business. You can share your customer's success stories via case studies, interviews, whitepapers or testimonials. This is known as social proof and one of the best forms of advertising that you could do for your business.

TIP: *A great way to interview your clients is to use a service called "Free Conference Call." It allows you to give* *your clients a number to call into and record the call. As the name states it is totally free. Once you have completed your interview with your client you can download it as an MP3 file.*

That MP3 file can be used on your website, used to put together a video, uploaded as a podcast, or used to build an email list of other interested clients.

This tip alone is well worth the price you paid for this book. That is a bulletproof way to increase your client base, and to build your name brand.

7. **Leverage the power of the holidays**

Holidays are also great opportunities to create some wonderful content by relating the holiday back to a product or service. You can also set-up a cool giveaway. After all who doesn't want a cool free gift around the holidays.

More Great Content Generating Ideas

You can literally get ideas for generating content from every day life. A good way to think out of the box is to use Google

Trends. This is another Google product that allows you to see what is trending in their search results.

NOTE: *Personally I stay away from politics and religion. It is a sure fire way to shoot yourself in the foot.*

Lets say that Google Trends happens to be trending something about a new movie release, you can ride on the coattails of that trend to generate a buzz about your business. For example, I knew that the movie Godzilla was going to be popular based on Google Trends. I had an article created for one of my sites entitled, "Godzilla VS Small Businesses". I was able to generate a massive amount of exposure for my services in a short time.

You can find ideas for generating content everywhere. Look for inspiration in everything that you do e.g. when you are watching your favorite television show, pay attention to commercials that you see. Look at advertisements on the side of the road, on YouTube, and in magazines.

Just because content isn't about your niche does not mean that you cannot generate ideas from it.

Jumpstarting Your SEO

Every business with a website should be trying to get the pages of their site ranked as high as possible in the search results. This is accomplished by applying specific SEO strategies. This should also be considered as part of your businesses growth strategy.

At its core, "SEO" is the methods used to increase your visibility in the search results. More exposure in the search results ultimately means more traffic to your website.

Before you start applying any SEO strategies to your website it is important to take a measurement and see where you are are at. This is a base. Without this you will have no idea if your efforts are working or not.

Where Are You Right Now?

You have no way of telling where you are as far as your marketing efforts, if you do not know where your website pages are currently ranked. Make sense? You will want to monitor your site closely. You want to know if it is moving up or down in the search results. You will want to know if your pages are being de-indexed.

Just to get a basic idea of where your site is ranked currently, you can either use Alexa, or Google toolbar. You will also want to check your site's referrer logs. This will allow you to track where your visitors are coming from. Your referrer logs will also tell you the search term that was used to find your site.

If you are clueless as to what I am talking about when I say "*check your referrer log*" check with your web hosting provider, who can tell you how to access the referrer logs for your site.

The Secrets To Using Keyword Phrases

Beware of where you are placing your keyword phrases throughout every aspect of your site e.g. Your titles, content, and even image names. It is a good idea to look at your keywords as search terms. Ask yourself, how would a prospect search for your products and or services. What would they type in to the search engine to find your page? The answer to that question is the keyword search phrase that you need to optimize a page on your site for.

For example, if your keyword research shows that people are searching for xyz widgets in Virginia Beach — you would want to optimize your page for that particular keyword phrase.

Your title tag and page header (*known as an H1 tag*) are the two most important areas to place your keyword phrases.

WARNING: I use to make the mistake of thinking this was obvious, and I neglected to mention it every time I was teaching. I would like to think that I learn from my mistakes. Take the following advice to heart, because if you do not I guarantee you that you will lose thousands of dollars.

So, here it goes:

Never… Ever… Place a ridiculous number of keywords on your web page. This is what is called "*spamming*" or "*keyword stuffing*". Please do not over do it!

Internal Linking Done Right

I cannot think of any other basic strategy as far as SEO is concerned than creating a well structured internal linking strategy for your website. You can easily accomplish this by implementing a plugin that I mentioned earlier entitled, "*Yet Another Related Post*".

Create A Sitemap

First let me start off by giving you a quick definition of what a sitemap is. It is a page that you generate that links to all the other major pages on your site. A site map makes it easier for search engine spiders to search and index your pages.

TIP: *If you are not already signed up for Google's Webmaster Tools, now would be a good time to do so.*

TO FLASH OR NOT TO FLASH

Sure Adobe Flash may look cool on your site, but it sucks for SEO. The internet marketing community has been arguing over the use of Adobe Flash, every since it was released in 2005.

If you ask 10 different SEO guru's if you should add Adobe Flash to your site I can guarantee you that you at least get a 50/50 split. I do not know about you, but I would not want the success or failure of my business coming down to a 50/50 split.

FACT: *Less than 82% of internet marketing companies do their own split testing to see what works and what does and does not work.*

My team and I have actually spent years testing using Adobe Flash in every way imaginable. The goal was to test the SEO pros and cons to using or not using Flash. Across the board Flash killed our search engine rankings.

It is my recommendation based on extensive testing that you avoid the use of Adobe Flash all together.

Optimizing Your Images

Search engine spiders only have the ability to search text, not text located in your images. This is why it is important to optimize your images with as much information as possible.

Start with your image name — you should "*always*" add an "*ALT*" tag which allows you to include a keyword rich description to your images.

EXAMPLE OF AN IMAGE ALT TAG

<img src="image.jpg" alt="your keyword phrase goes here along with description">

Optimizing your images is just another way that you can gain that cutting edge over your competitors. When it comes to online marketing you want to take advantage of every possible resource.

Something as simple as using the **bold**, or *italic* feature in your content could make the difference between being ranked 1 or 2 in the search engines.

Anticipating Your Prospects Next Move

I was sitting in my home office one day when my son came in and asked me to play a video game called Guitar Hero. With a smile on his face, he looked at me and said:

"You can go first dad. I am going to set the game on easy mode for you to give you a chance."

I am sitting there with this toy guitar in my hand, waiting for the game to begin. Colorful dots began flying across the screen and I have to perfectly coordinate pressing the buttons on the guitar with the dots that appear on the screen. I must admit that it did give me the feeling of being a real rock star. Before you knew it my game was over and my score flashed across the screen. I was feeling pretty good about my score if I must say so myself. I looked at my son and reminded him that I was the Pac-Man, Space Invader, and Donkey Kong champ back in the day.

It was now his turn. He put the game on expert mode, and selected his song. I was amazed at how fast the little dots were flying across the screen. What amazed me even more is that he was able to trash talk to me while he was playing the game. Finally his turn was over and he placed the guitar down and extended his hand to shake mine. The gloating went on for several minutes.

If you have a child or a niece or nephew, chances are you have experienced this same thing.

My son was so good at this video game because he has played it over and over again. He knows everything that is going to happen before it happens.

This same principal applies to your online marketing. You do not want to react to what is currently happing, you want to anticipate what is going to happen. It is always best to be ahead of the curve, rather than behind the curve.

If I asked you, "*would you be interested in increasing your profits, what would you say?*"

Your answer would be yes of course. One of your primary motivations for being in business is to generate a profit. Let's say that last year you generated 100 sales, and or transactions. If I could show you how to increase this years sales by 10% with an extremely low investment and spending less than 30 minutes a week to get it to work, would you be interested?

Again, your answer would be yes. It's a no-brainer.

Because of my reputation, most business owners expect me to come in and give them some magical solution that will increase their profits. They are shocked when I tell them that before thinking outside of the box, I want to get the resources inside of the box organized.

"99% of companies have money that they are leaving on the table."

When I consult for a client, it is my job to first and foremost make changes from within. I already know upfront, it is going to be like pulling teeth. As human beings we are predisposed to change.

Before we talk about implementing any changes lets first make sure that we are on the same page.

There are only three ways to grow any business no matter what it is. It doesn't matter if you are an army of one working from the comforts of your kitchen table or you are a multi-billion dollar organization. Here are the only three ways to grow your business:

1. Increase number of visitors.
2. Increase number of transactions.
3. Increase cost per transaction.

That's it! Nothing magical about it.

The GateKeeper

Trust me when I tell you that the gatekeeper knows everything that is going on in your organization. In most businesses the gatekeeper only answers the phones, and takes messages. What a waste of a valuable resource.

I am blown away at how many times I hear a gatekeeper answer the phone like this.

GateKeeper: "Hello, XYZ Company how may I help you?"

Caller: "Yes I was looking for information about your abc service?"

GateKeeper: "Excellent, I can help you with that."

The gatekeeper will then go on to answer the callers questions and that is it.

Take a look at the way the call should be handled:

GateKeeper: "Hello, XYZ Company how may I help you?"

Caller: "Yes I was looking for information about your abc service?"

GateKeeper: "Excellent, I can help you with that. By the way, if you do not mind me asking, how did you hear about us?"

That last question is the key. The gatekeeper should always ask the caller how did they hear about your company "*before*" they move on to helping the caller.

Something as simple as the question, "*How did you hear about us*" will give you statistical information that is extremely valuable to your marketing efforts. Lets say that you are running ads on the radio, television, online, and in your local newspaper. By asking the caller how did they hear about you, would allow you to gather crucial statistical data. Lets say that you discovered that 70% of your leads were coming from the Internet. 5% of your leads were coming from radio, 20% from television, and another 5% from the newspaper. Do you think that information would help you make better decisions on how to spend your advertising dollars?

Of course it would!

The best part about this strategy is that it will only cost you the price of a pen and paper. Your tracking method doesn't have to be anything fancy. There is no need to invest hundreds of dollars on useless software.

At the end of each day have the gatekeeper email, or leave the results on your desk to look over.

By implementing this simple tactic you can easily figure out where to invest your marketing dollars. You now know what is working and what needs to be improved or eliminated.

Often times we hear business owners claim that they are already doing this. However further research reveals more often than not that this strategy is not being implemented on a consistent basis. By being inconsistent, you are skewing the data and you will not have factual information to base your marketing decisions on.

By being armed with the right information you will have the ability to anticipate where your prospects are spending their time, and what type of marketing your prospects respond to best. This will allow you to increase your website's visitors (*method number one to growing a business*).

YouTube VS Television

Select someone from your office that is knowledgable about your business and make them the spokes person. Create videos that consist of advice and tips that will appeal to your prospects.

Create a YouTube channel for your niche market. Schedule regular video posts. If you decide to post videos every Monday, make sure that you post every Monday without fail.

You can leverage the content that you create for your YouTube channel by using it on your website. Your YouTube content can also be posted to your social media accounts e.g. Twitter, Facebook, LinkedIn, and Google+.

TIP: *You do not need expensive camera equipment to make good videos. You can use any smart device to get the job done. Depending on your lighting situation you may want to pick up a few garage lights with stands from your local Lowes or Home Depot.*

Always plan out your videos first. You should have at least an outline of what material is going to be covered.

Once you have your blueprint you can shoot all of your videos at one time.

Most small to medium size businesses are not using this type of strategy to generate new prospects. By implementing a video marketing strategy you will have a huge advantage over and above the competition. It will be easy for you to become the leading authority in your market space. As with any other form of marketing you have to be consistent.

More Americans watch videos on YouTube than they do television. As a savvy business owner you want to anticipate where your prospects will be next. Do you think that YouTube would be a good bet? Of course it would. The writing is on the wall, all you have to do is follow it.

How Business Cards Can Increase Your Business

Every business book on earth will tell you the old mumbo-jumbo about getting business cards etc. I'm not going to rehash what you already know. Besides getting business cards alone will not do anything for you. In fact most business cards end up sitting on a shelf or they end up stuffed in a drawer somewhere.

Of course I have a strategy that will help bring in extra business without a lot of effort. This strategy has been sitting under your nose all the time but you have not been using it.

Get your employees business cards, with a title "*work*" phone number, and your website address. Offer the employees a little incentive for every lead that you close.

Let's take a look at what I call employee psychology. Even if you do not want to admit it, your employees do not have a stake in your company "yet". If you succeed or fail, they really do not care. If you were to go out of business today, your employees would get another job and continue collecting a paycheck.

However, if you were to give them a little incentive, such as a bonus, your employees would have a reason to go out and promote your business.

I have a service that I sell for $400 a month. I have a team that makes cold calls in order to sell my service. For each person that signs up, my team member will receive $150 for the life of the client.

One of my team members is a single mother of three who made 7 sales the first month of cold calling. The second month she only made 3 sales. The third month she made a whopping 10 sales. I cut her a check every month for $3,000. I will continue cutting her a check as long as the customer continues paying.

Do you think your employees will be more motivated if there was some type of incentive? Again the answer is yes.

Increase Your Leads With Two Words

I know you're probably thinking, "*come on now, there is no way that I can increase my leads with two words.*" Well let me explain myself. The words, "*thank you*" will open up a lot of doors for you. Start with the clients that have already done business with you.

Although you should already have a list of clients and their contact information, I am going to start from scratch as if you just opened the doors today.

From this point on you will want to gather as much information as possible about your clients, and prospects. Drop them a thank you card.

Let's say that you have a prospect call and ask you about your services. Ask them if they mind giving you their email address to send them any specials or updates that you may have. Once they give it to you, ask for their phone number (*that's called an embedded command and they will follow your instructions on autopilot*).

If they do not decide to come in for a consultation, shoot them a thank you email. Your email should go something like this:

Hey John,

Thank you for giving us a call regarding our services. Although you did not schedule a consultation this time. I will be calling you soon to see if you may have changed your mind.

Thanks
YOUR NAME

TIP: *When sending a physical "Thank You" card it should be handwritten. If you try to print it — it increases the odds of your thank you card not getting read.*

I do not recommend you using my exact wording. Change it up and make it your own. The most important thing to remember is to follow up with your client as you promised. I personally use thank you cards for all aspects of my life.

There is this nice little restaurant that I have been frequenting for years. After all of this time I still send them thank you cards for their outstanding service. I send a thank you card to the manager, and to the head office. When I go there to have lunch with a client, trust me I receive better service than the president would if he were to walk in.

I do the same at the Mercedes dealership, the gym, and even my neighborhood dry cleaners. Business owners often forget the power of the simple words, thank you.

How To Become A Master At Anticipating

Anticipation is like a muscle. The more that you exercise it, the stronger it will become. Just like any muscle that you exercise, it will take a conscious effort to improve it. With practice, your ability to anticipate will become second nature. You will have the ability to size up your options and possible responses that will lead you to your desired outcome.

Here are 4 strategies that will help you increase your anticipation muscle:

1. Know your business inside and out. Know who your direct competitors are. Our ability to anticipate is birthed out of knowledge and the skill of leveraging that knowledge towards a desired result.

2. Start training yourself to think in "*what ifs*'." Train yourself along with your employees to consider the relationship of cause and effect in every decision that they make. Practice thinking through scenarios with a "*What if we did ___*" or "*What if we responded like ___*" and then consider the effect each might bring. Consider how each decision that you make impacts the next decision. By applying this simple strategy you will develop a great perspective that will enable future anticipation to become automatic whenever similar scenarios unfold.

3. Slow down and think it through. Way to often we get caught up in the day-to-day routine and we make hasty decisions. If we are speeding through the day we will miss the ability to capitalize on a strategic choices. In the words of the late great Zig Ziglar, give yourself a checkup from the neck up randomly throughout the day. Take inventory or your surroundings and ask yourself are you being observant? If not, start paying attention, and keep your eyes open for opportunity.

4. Being aware is one of the best ways to anticipate. Evaluate your choices then act. If you were sitting at a 4-way intersection and saw someone else approaching at a rapid speed, you would likely anticipate that the other driver isn't about to stop. You could only see that if you were aware and paying attention. If you were messing with your radio, or cell phone or otherwise distracted, you might roll through the intersection and get t-boned.

Practice the above strategies in all aspects of your life. Before you know it you will be making masterful decisions concerning your business.

Increase Your Leads

At this point in the guide you clearly understand that your website is like a teacher/sales person that represents your company 24/7. Generating exposure and generating traffic is only part of the battle. Sure getting traffic to your website is a great accomplishment, however it is nothing if you do not know how to get that traffic to convert.

Better Call To Action

Your call to action should be above the fold. When I say above the fold I am talking about the space viewable to the user without having to scroll down. According to heat map analysis research, anything that is below the fold will only be viewed by 50% of the website visitors who view the page.

Clarity Is Key

I cannot begin to tell you how many times I have visited a website that was trying to make an offer, but I had no clue exactly what it was they were offering. It is your goal to be crystal clear. If you are offering a free ebook, say something like "*Download our FREE ebook on how to ___*". If you are offering a discount say something along the lines of, "*Register here to receive $100 off*". The point is you should clearly convey a compelling benefit of receiving the offer.

Images VS Text

Take a look at your list of competitor sites that I told you to write down in the beginning. Check to see how many of them have a visible CTA. Also look to see how many of them use an image to make their CTA standout.

I am sure you have heard the saying that an image is worth a thousand words. Studies have proven that using an image for your CTA converts better than plain text.

If at all possible place your CTA offer above the fold and on as many pages as possible.

Conflicting Colors On Your Site

Ok, this next one is going to cause problems. Your web designer is going to kick and scream about this, but it has to be done. If the color of your CTA blends in with your web site design the visitor will just pass it by. You want your CTA to pop off the page. Do not be afraid to test different things and get creative with it.

Creating Landing Pages That Convert

At this point you should have your CTA set and ready to go. The page that your CTA will link to is called a landing page. You will want to make sure that the headline of your landing page matches your CTA offer. This ties everything together.

When the visitor clicks on your CTA and hit your landing page you want them to know that they are in the right place. Keep your message consistent on both your CTA offer and your landing pages.

If you are offering them a free download, or some sort of coupon, you better do as you say. If you lose the trust of your prospects the bad news will spread. When customers and prospects are upset, or frustrated it only takes a few mouse clicks to spread slanderous information about your business. That could easily cost you thousands of dollars. The best strategy is to deliver more than you promise. A happy customer is a customer that will recommend others.

Keep Your Form Simple

I am amazed at how many people have these long complicated forms on their site. Then they sit back with a silly look on their face and wonder why the form is not converting.

When creating your form, you should only ask for what you need to convert the prospect.

Just like with your CTA you will want to have your form at the top of the fold. You do not want the prospect to have to scroll in order to find your form. You will want to also make the form pop off the page. You will want your form to grab the users attention right away.

Creating Copy For Your Landing Pages

Be brief and to the point; it's the offer where you give the prospect more information. In addition to your headline, have a brief paragraph explaining what the offer is, followed by a few bullet points outlining what the offer consists of and what the benefits are.

Make it clear in your brief paragraph and/or bullet points what the benefits of the offer are. It's more than just listing what the offer is comprised of; it takes a bit of spin. Instead of "*includes specs of about product xyz*", say something like "*Find out how xyz can increase your profits by 25%*".

When a prospect reaches your landing page, you're just a few keystrokes away from getting their contact information. So don't distract them with links that will take them further away from your goal of getting a lead. The thank you page, shown after a prospect fills out a form and becomes a lead, will give you the opportunity to return the navigation and links.

When creating a thank you page, not only can you give back the navigation, but you can provide other links to keep the lead engaged. You can provide call to actions to the next step in the buying cycle, link them to your blog, encourage them to follow you on a social media site, ask them to subscribe to your newsletter, and more. Just note that you should use your landing page as an opportunity to further engage your prospect.

Making Your Offer Irresistible

Ok, brace yourself. I am about to be brutally honest with you. So, this may sting a little. Prospects do not give a damn about you or your business. All they want to know is, "*what's in it for them!*"

This is why your offer should immediately answer their biggest question. Things such as pricing brochures, specs, and self-promotional videos are not compelling offers. They do not answer the prospects burning question. Informational items like whitepapers, guides, and webinars are a few compelling offers because it lets the prospect know exactly what is in it for them. Do you see the difference?

When you are making your offer immediately go for the knock out blow. Tell the client right off what is in it for them. Tell them how they will benefit from using your products and or services.

Your Reputation Can Make or Break Your Business

What people have to say about your business online has become the single most important reflection of your business's quality, reliability, and skill. It does not matter if you are a hair transplant clinic, plastic surgeon, plumber, or you are in the home health care industry. When it comes to doing business in the digital age — reality means nothing and perception means everything.

In Nielsen's most recent Global Trust in Advertising study, 70% of global consumers indicated they trust online reviews from strangers when making purchasing decisions.

You have sacrificed blood, sweat and tears to build your business. As you reflect back on how and where everything started, you start to feel a sense of accomplishment. You feel as if it's time to reap the benefits of all your hard work.

Out of the blue a client walks in and mentions a negative review that he or she seen posted online. You read the review and disagree with it. You continue on with life. Then you start to notice that business has slowed down. The calls are not coming in the way that they use to. Your website leads have dried up. Sounds like a nightmare doesn't it? This is a sad case, but it is something that is happening to thousands of businesses across the country.

The reputation of your business is an extremely important part of doing business in the digital age. I find it heartbreaking that many business owners are taking their online reputation lightly.

What business owners do not understand is that a negative online reputation can bankrupt a business. The internet allows people to hide behind their computer screens and say whatever they want to. Any negative thing that is said about your business could be harmful, even if it is not true. It is not always a client that posts negative reviews. Many competitors and disgruntle employees will post negative reviews also.

One of your top marketing priorities should be developing a stellar online reputation. Your reputation is the lynchpin to all of your other marketing efforts. If you have a horrible reputation it will drive prospects away from you and into the arms of your competitors.

When a prospect does a search for a local business, even though at first glance the words from a negative review may not show up, your ratings will in the form of a five star rating system.

You could work hard to get your business ranked number one in the search results, but a poor rating will make a prospect skip your listing and go to the one with the higher rating.

Consumers want information that will help them to feel confident that they are making the best decision. In the digital age, the consumers confidence comes in the form of online reviews which in the eyes of the consumer reflects the experiences of others like them.

FACT: Consumers will trust the words of others that they deem to be like them before they trust any words coming from a business owner.

The 5 Pillars To Building A Positive Online Reputation

Before you dive in and start developing, building, and protecting your online reputation, you need to commit these five points to memory:

1. **Range** - Do not count on a few resources for your reviews. Although Yelp, and Google are important, there are dozens of others out there that you should take into consideration as well.

2. **Real** - It is your job to ensure that real client reviews are getting posted. Scrupulous businesses have tried to game the system by posting rave reviews. This is not only unethical, you will sooner or later have to face the music. These sites

are getting better and better at finding fake reviews. You should Encourage your customers to be as specific as possible when posting a review about your business.

3. **Recent** - Google's algorithm is constantly changing. This means that I can only share with you information that is working at this time. It would appear that Google gives some credibility in terms of rankings. This is an excellent reason to create a steady flow of new, positive reviews. It is important to note that more recent reviews have more weight, and social proof with prospects versus older reviews.

4. **Quantity** - If a doctor had 30 reviews with a 4-star average and the next best has one 5-star review, who would you do business with? Reliability is proven with consistency, particularly where reviews are concerned.

5. **Quality -** I would like to think that this one is pretty obvious. The higher the reviews, the better your status

will be - within reason. A business with nothing but a 5-star rating can look suspicious, but in general, the more favorable your reviews, the better.

How To Charge More And Make Your Customers Thank You

By now you should understand that your business "*must*" put a reputation building process in place. The time and investment that you make right now will be well worth the benefits. There is one more little hidden secret to having a top notch rating and it's called — pricing power.

If you have been in business for any length of time you know what it feels like to have to defend your prices. Imagine how easy it would be to respond to the question, "*Why should I pay more for your product/service?*" All you have to say is, "*Have you taken a look online to see what our clients are saying?*"

Businesses need to leverage the power a 5-star reputation brings. You've worked hard to establish your business and sacrificed plenty along the way. The million dollar question is, "*Are you willing to let that hard work get flushed down the drain because of a single disgruntled client or competitor?*"

The Future of Marketing Is Here

Marketing at its core is all about getting the most targeted exposure for your business as humanly possible. The more pages you have indexed in Google the more you increase the odds of people visiting your site.

Exposure, Exposure, Exposure

For a physical business the most important concern is, location, location, location. For a business online the number one rule is exposure, exposure, exposure.

Do a search for any industry keyword phrase. Chances are you will see Yelp, Wikipedia, Yellow Pages, or some similar site.

Do you know why these sites dominate the search results for nearly everything that you search for? Its because they are power houses of content, and they have straight forward page structures.

Most businesses do not have the ability nor the resources to create a massive amount of content. This makes it difficult for the little guy to compete. Since most business owners do not understand that they have lost the battle before they even had a chance, they continue dumping thousands of dollars into a internet marketing campaign that they simply cannot win. This is a growing problem that I have spent most of my career trying to solve.

Early 2012 we had what we felt was the ultimate solution. We dove right in and started testing our concept in a variety of niche markets on my personal sites.

We were literally dominating the search results. The entire team was extremely excited. We thought it was to good to be true. Then Google began their rounds of updates. As always after Google's update business owners were yelling and screaming about losing search engine rankings.

Our marketing project withstood Google's major updates. The way business owners market online will never be the same once we release our new marketing methods for local businesses.

What Does This Mean For You

We will go out and build a geo-targeted network in your niche market (*this doesn't cost you anything*). We get the pages from our network indexed in Google. I'm talking about thousands of pages. Once we get the pages indexed we will point them towards your site using our new technology. That means "*instantly*" we can point thousands of pages towards any page you choose from your domain.

Here's How It Works

We build a huge network in your niche market. The content on the network would be based on geo-targeted keyword phrases (*e.g. hair loss specialist in youngstown ohio*) for every city and state in the United States. The network will be rented out by states.

Once you rent out any available state, my team and I will continue to build out our network which means your exposure will continue to grow.

The best part is no matter how much the network grows, your cost stays the same.

If you would like to see an actual demo give us a call - 757-271-5605.

Things To Do Before You Call

- Please be sitting in front of a computer with an internet connection.
- In order to save time you will need to know how many pages you currently have indexed. You can find this out by entering the following into Google: site:yourdomain.com - you will need to know the approximate number of pages that you currently have indexed. You can find the number right under the search bar.

- Give us a call and prepare to be amazed - 757-271-5605.

Final Words

Congratulations, you have completed reading this book. The information that you have gained is worthless if you do not implement it.

According to the godfather of modern day business, business is 90% marketing, and 10% inspiration.

Some say that knowledge is power. It is my belief that knowledge is potential power. No matter how much knowledge you possess if you fail to do anything with it your knowledge is useless.

Do not let the knowledge that you have learned in this guide go to waste. Start implementing the strategies today.

I will end this guide with my definition of marketing:

Marketing *- the act of increasing the exposure for your business, product(s) and or service(s) in hopes of increasing your leads, sales and ultimately your companies bottom line.*

Glossary of Internet Marketing Terms

301 Redirect – A 301 redirect automatically causes one url to redirect to another and tells the Web (*and search engines*) that this redirect is permanent, as opposed to a temporary (*302*) redirect. 301 redirects are generally preferable for Search Engine Optimization purposes and are therefore often referred to as search engine friendly redirects.

404 Server Code – The 404 or Not Found error message is a standard response code indicating that the client was able to communicate with a given server, but the server could not find what was requested.

Above the Fold – The part of the page you can see without scrolling down or over. The exact amount of space will vary by viewer because of screen settings. You often pay a premium for advertisement placements above the fold, which will add to the costs of internet marketing services, but may also add to results.

adCenter – Microsoft adCenter powers paid search results on Microsoft's bing, Yahoo! (*as of November 2010*), and other sites within its network. Microsoft adCenter is now the second largest paid search provider in the United States.

Advertising Network – A group of websites where one advertiser controls all or a portion of the ads for all sites. A common example is the Google Search Network, which includes AOL, Amazon, Ask.com (*formerly Ask Jeeves*), and thousands of other sites. In Google AdWords, they offer two types of ad networks on the internet: search and display (*which used to be called their content network*).

AdWords – AdWords is Google's paid search marketing program, the largest such program in the world and in most countries with notable exceptions such as China (*Baidu*) and Russia (*Yandex*). Introduced in 2001, AdWords was the first pay per click provider offering the concept of Quality Score, factoring search relevancy (*via click-through rate*) in along with bid to determine ad position.

Affiliate Marketing – A type of internet marketing in which you partner with other websites, individuals, or companies to send traffic to your site. You will typically pay on a *Cost per Acquisition (CPA)* or *Cost per Click (CPC)* basis.

Algorithm – The term search engines use for the formulae they use to determine the rankings of your *Natural Listings*. Search engines will periodically send a spider/bot through your website to view all its information. Their programs (*bots)* analyze your sites data to value your site and fix whether or not, and how high or low pages on your site will appear on various searches. These algorithms can be very complicated (*Google alone currently uses 106 different variables*) and search engines closely guard their algorithms as trade secrets.

ALT Tags – HTML tags used to describe website graphics by displaying a block of text when moused-over. Search engines are generally unable to view graphics or distinguish text that might be contained within them, and the implementation of an ALT tag enables search engines to categorize that graphic. There is also talk that business websites will all be required to utilize ALT tags for all pictures to comply with certain American Disability Act requirements.

Analytics– Also known as Web Metrics. Analytics refers to a collection of data about a website and its users. Analytics programs typically give performance data on clicks, time, pages viewed, website paths, and a variety of other information. The proper use of Web analytics allows website owners to improve their visitor experience, which often leads to higher ROI for profit-based sites.

Anchor Text – The clickable words of a *hypertext link*; they will appear as the underlined blue part in standard Web design. In the preceding sentence, "*hypertext link*" is the anchor text. As with anything in SEO, it can be overdone, but generally speaking, using your important keywords in the anchor text is highly desirable.

Astroturfing – The process of creating fake grassroots campaigns. Astroturfing is often used specifically regarding review sites like Google Places, Yelp, Judy's Book and more. These fake reviews can be positive reviews for your own company or slander against your competitors. Not a good idea, and could lead to your IP being blacklisted. The worse case scenario is a lawsuit.

Backlinks– Links from other websites pointing to any particular page on your site. Search engines use backlinks to judge a site's credibility; if a site links to you, the reasoning goes, it is in effect vouching for your authority on a particular subject. Therefore, Link Building is an incredibly important part of Search Engine Optimization. How many links, the quality of the sites linking to you, and how they link to you all are important factors. Also called *Inbound Links*.

Baidu– Serving primarily China, Baidu is the largest non-US based search engine in the world (*although it was started in the United States*). Sites can be optimized for Baidu and they offer their own paid search service.

Banned – When pages are removed from a search engine's index specifically because the search engine has deemed them to be violating their guidelines. Although procedures are starting to loosen up somewhat, typically a search engine will not confirm to you that your site has been banned or why it has been banned. If you knowingly did something against the rules (*written or unwritten*) that got your site banned, you can probably clean up your act and get back in the game. We hear stories that, from time to time of companies hiring Search Engine Optimization companies that deliver great, fast results, leave town, and then their website mysteriously disappears from the rankings. Google won't tell them why their site got banned, so the company ends up left out in the cold unless another company can come in and backwards engineer the issues, unravel the work, and get the search engine to reinclude the site.

Banners – Picture advertisements placed on websites. Such advertising is often a staple of internet marketing branding campaigns. Depending upon their size and shape, banner ads may also be referred to as buttons, inlines, leaderboards, skyscrapers, or other terms. When using specifics, banner ads refer to a 468×60 pixel size. Banner ads can be static pictures, animated, or interactive. Banner ads appear anywhere on a site – top, middle, bottom, or side. Banner costs vary by website and advertiser; two of the most popular pay structures are Cost per 1,000 Impressions (*CPM*) and flat costs for a specified period of time.

Behavioral Targeting (BT) – An area of internet marketing becoming increasingly refined, behavioral targeting looks to put ads in front of people who should be more receptive to the particular message given past Web behavior, including purchases and websites visited. The use of cookies enables online behavioral targeting.

Bing – Bing is Microsoft's search engine, which replaced live.com in June 2009. Bing results now power Yahoo!'s search for paid (*except display; through Microsoft adCenter*) and organic (*except local listings*) through an alliance entered into between the two Web giants in December 2009. The deal cleared regulatory concerns in early 2010 and was fully completed in November of the same year.

Black Hat SEO – The opposite of White Hat SEO, these Search Engine Optimization, or SEO, tactics are (*attempted*) ways of tricking the Search Engines to get better rankings for a website. If not immediately, using black hat methods will eventually get your site drastically lower rankings or banned from the search engines altogether. While there are completely legal and ethical techniques you can use to improve rankings, if you design and market a website mostly for humans and not for the search engines' you should be okay.

Blog – Short for Web log, blogs are part journal, part website. Typically the newest entry (*blog post*) appears at the top of the page with older entries coming after in reverse chronological order. Several blogging platforms exist; our favorite is WordPress.

Brand Stacking – Multiple page one listings from a single domain. Prior to 2010, a site would be fortunate if it had three first page results for branded searches. Since Google tweaked its algorithm to include Brand Stacking, that number has risen to as many as eight of the top search rankings.

Categories – Words or phrases used to organize blog posts and other pieces of information, such as albums for photos. Categories are generally broader than tags and used in instances when there will generally be multiple posts or other data points per category.

ccTLD – ccTLD's are "Country-code" *TLD's* showing what country a site is focused on or based in. Using Google and the United Kingdom as an example, Google UK is google.co.uk. Sometimes

these ccTLD's are two sets of letters separated by a period (*e.g. "co.uk" for the UK or "com.au" for Australia*) and sometimes they are just one set of letters (*e.g. ".fr" for France*).
Use of separate websites on unique ccTLD's is typically viewed as the best way for exporters to target other countries via search engine optimization. However, site owners can also target outside countries through other means such as through country-focused subdomains or even subdirectories.

Click through Rate (CTR) – # of clicks / # of impressions. Click through rate is a common internet marketing measurement tool for ad effectiveness. This rate tells you how many times people are actually clicking on your ad out of the number of times your ad is shown. Low click through rates can be caused by a number of factors, including copy, placement, and relevance.

Cloaking– Showing a search engine spider or bot one version of a Web page and a different version to the end user.

Several search engines have explicit rules against unapproved cloaking. Those violating these guidelines may find their pages penalized or banned from a search engine's index. As for approved cloaking, this generally only happens with search engines that offer a paid inclusion program. Anyone offering cloaking services should be able to demonstrate explicit approval from a search engine for what it is they intend to do.

Content Management System – Content Management Systems (*CMS*) allow website owners to make text and picture changes to their websites without specialized programming knowledge of software like Adobe Dreamweaver or Microsoft FrontPage. Content Management Systems can be edited by anyone with basic word knowledge via an internet connection. No need for length or costly web development contracts or need to wait on someone outside your company to make changes. CMS examples include WordPress, Drupal, and Joomla.

Content Network – Each major search engine offers a form of content network within its paid search interface, typically referred to as content networks, although Google just renamed their content network the Google Display Network. Within Google AdWords, advertisers have two options for content network advertising:

1. *Pick sites.* With this option, you can choose the actual sites, or in some cases, sections and pages of sites, on which you want to display your ads.

2. *Contextual advertising.* Contextual advertising allows you to use keywords like you would in traditional paid search advertising and the search engines will display your ads next to articles, blog posts, and other Web pages that are related to those keywords.

Both options are great for inexpensive brand awareness on massive scales in addition to more direct means such as lead generation. The days of buying remnant display ads not being worth it are behind us.

Content Tags – HTML tags which define the essence of the content contained within them and readable by search spiders. These include Header and Alt Tags.

Contextual Advertising – A feature offered by major search engine advertisers allowing your advertisement to be placed next to related news articles and on other Web pages. Contextual advertising seeks to match Web content from the display page with your advertised search term(s). Contextual advertising isn't perfect (*what in life is?*), but it's come a long way from its inception to the point where it can provide great value to advertisers when used correctly.

Conversion Rate – This statistic, or metric, tells you what percentage of people is converting (*really!*). The definition of "conversion" depends upon your goals and measurements. It could mean a sign up for free information, a completed survey, a purchase made, or other.

Cookie – Think of cookies like Batman's Bat Tracer. When you visit a website, Batman sticks a cookie on your browser to follow you around. Batman can then go back to his Bat Cave and watch where you're going and where you've been. A little Big Brother-ish to be sure, but cookies also provide direct benefits to surfers, including remembering passwords and bringing you offers in which you are genuinely interested (see Behavioral Targeting above).

Cost per Acquisition (CPA) – An online advertising cost structure where you pay per an agreed upon actionable event, such as a lead, registration, or sale.

Cost per Click (CPC) – A common way to pay for search engine and other types of online advertising, CPC means you pay a pre-determined amount each time someone clicks on your advertisement to visit your site. You usually set a top amount you are willing to pay per click for each search term, and the amount you pay will be equal or less to that amount, depending on the particular search engine and your competitors' bids. Also referred to as Pay Per Click (*PPC*) or Paid Search Marketing.

Cost per Impression (CPM) – A common internet marketing cost structure, especially for banner advertising. You agree to pay a set cost for every 1,000 Impressions your ad receives. Search engine marketing may involve CPM costs for Contextual Advertising. This internet advertising pay structure should really be called Cost per 1,000 Impressions.

Crawler – Component of a search engine that gathers listings by automatically "crawling" the Web. A search engine's crawler (also known as a Spider or robot) follows links to Web Pages. It makes copies of those pages and stores them in a search engine's index.

CSS – CSS – short for Cascading Style Sheet – is a way to move style elements off individual Web pages and sites to allow for faster loading pages, smaller file sizes, and other benefits for visitors, search engines, and designers.

Customer Relationship Management (CRM) – Software solutions that help enterprise businesses manage customer relationships in an organized way. An example of a CRM would be a database containing detailed customer information that management and salespeople can reference in order to match customer needs with products, inform customers of service requirements, etc.

Day Parting – Day parting refers to serving ads at different times of the day and days of the week, or even changing bids or copy / creative at different times. For example, you may not want your ads to show from 11AM-2PM on Tuesdays. This can be done manually in most online platforms, or automatically in some such as Google AdWords. Automated day parting is not currently available directly through many social media advertising platforms such as facebook ads and LinkedIn direct ads.

Delisting – When pages or whole websites are removed from a search engine's index. This may happen because, but not necessarily, they have been Banned.

Description Tags – HTML tags which provide a brief description of your site that search engines can understand. Description tags should contain the main keywords of the page it is describing in a short summary – don't go crazy here with Keyword Stuffing.

Directories – A type of search engine where listings are gathered through human efforts rather than Web crawling. In directories, websites are often reviewed, summarized to a brief description and placed in a relevant category.

Domain Name – A website's main address. 4th Generation Communication's domain is www.4thgc.com.

Doorway Page – A Web page created to rank well in a search engine's organic listings (*non-paid*) and delivers very little information to those viewing it. Instead, visitors will often only see a brief call to action (*i.e., "Click Here to Enter"*), or they may be automatically propelled past the doorway page. With cloaking, they may never see the doorway page at all. Several search engines have guidelines against doorway pages, though they are more commonly allowed through paid inclusion programs. Also referred to as bridge pages, gateway pages and jump pages and not to be confused with Landing Pages.

Domain Name Monitoring – Watching Domains across various extensions. Some companies offer to do this for, say a .com site by checking the same domain name in .net, .org, .eu, etc.

eCommerce – The ability to purchase online. eCommerce also goes by other super-snazzy names like etail. website features that allow ecommerce are commonly called shopping carts.

EdgeRank – The algorithm facebook uses to rank a page's or profile's posts to determine which of those posts will appear in the newsfeeds of users connected to those pages and profiles (*or pages and profiles tagged in the posts*). The higher an EdgeRank, the more likely you will appear in the newsfeeds. Facebook does not release this data publicly, neither for the pages, nor individual posts.

Ego Keyword – A keyword an individual or organization feels it must rank for in either or both *natural listings* or *paid search results* regardless of cost and *Return on Investment*. Read more about ego keywords.

Email Campaign System – Email is perhaps the most overlooked and underutilized (based on cost and effectiveness) form of internet marketing today. Email campaign systems allow organizations to send out emails to their email lists with a standard look and feel. Features often include the ability to segment lists.

Enhanced Bidding – A feature specific to Google AdWords. When you select to utilize enhanced bidding, you're giving

AdWords the power to adjust your bidding in order to increase conversions. With this feature, you can pay up to 30% over the keyword bid that you set. Think of it like a hybrid between CPC and CPA bidding, albeit still more heavily weighted toward cost per click. Be careful with enhanced bidding – many search engine marketers will tell you that they have had poor experiences with cost per acquisition bidding within AdWords.

Eyetracking – A process that allows testing of websites for usability or any other purpose. Eyetracking is performed by a small number of companies utilizing high speed cameras to monitor and record where the eyes of test subjects actually move on screen.

Facebook Retargeting – While this term can also refer to other forms of retargeting, it is most often used to mean serving ads to prior site visitors while those visitors are on facebook. Facebook opened its ad exchange in December 2012 to allow partners to offer facebook retargeting.

Feed – Coming in an XML language that uses either *RSS* or Atom formatting are an extremely popular way for organizations to get their messages through the clutter and into the hands of interested parties. With the simple click of an orange button (*right*), users can stay connected to a site's content (*Blogs, news, podcasts, etc.*) automatically anytime their computers are connected to the internet. That button will connect you to the feed for the Found Blog.

Forum – A place on the internet where people with common interests or backgrounds come together to find information and discuss topics.

Geo-Targeting – The ability to reach potential clients by their physical location. The major search engines now all offer the ability to geo-target searches in their *Pay-Per-Click* campaigns by viewing their ip addresses. Geo-targeting allows advertisers to specify which markets they do and don't want to reach.

Golden Triangle - Eye-tracking studies show an "F" shaped pattern that most people tend to look at most often when looking at Search Engine Results Pages. These patterns vary slightly among the different Search Engines, but show the importance of placement among Natural Listings and Pay-per-Click ads.

Google AdWords Certified Partner – Google AdWords offers the most extensive certification process of any of the paid search marketing providers. The Google AdWords Certified Partner program replaces the earlier Qualified Google Advertising Company / Individual program.

Graphical Search Inventory – Banners and other types of advertising units which can be synchronized to search keywords. Includes pop-ups browser toolbars and rich media.

Header (or Heading) Tags () – HTML heading and subheading tags are critical components of search engine marketing, as often times both are graphical, thereby unreadable to search engine spiders. Optimally, page titles should also be included to clearly define the page's purpose and theme. All of the header tags should be used according to their relevance, with more prominent titles utilizing <h1>, subheaders using <h2>, and so on.

HTML– HyperText Markup Language, the programming language used in websites. Developers use other languages that can be read and understood by HTML to expand what they can do on the Web.

Hyperlink – Often blue and underlined, hyperlinks, commonly called "links" for short, allow you to navigate to other pages on the Web with a simple click of your mouse.

Image Maps – Clickable regions on images that make links more visually appealing and websites more interesting. Image maps enable spiders to "*read*" this material.

Impressions – The number of times someone views a page displaying your ad. Note that this is not the same as actually seeing your ad, making placement and an understanding of the site's traffic particularly important when paying on a Cost per 1,000 Impressions basis.

Inbound or Incoming Links – See Backlinks

Index – The collection of information a search engine has that searchers can query against. With crawler-based search engines, the index is typically copies of all the Web pages they have found from crawling the Web. With human-powered directories, the index contains the summaries of all the websites that have been categorized.

Internet Marketing – Any of a number of ways to reach internet users, including Search Engine Marketing, Search Engine Optimization, and Banner advertising. Direct Online Marketing™ specializes in these internet marketing services.

Internal Linking – Placing hyperlinks on a page to other pages *within the same* *site*. This helps users find more information, improve site interaction, and enhances your SEO efforts.

Interstitial – An ad that appears between two pages a person is trying to view. The ad often appears near a hyperlink allowing someone to quit viewing your ad and go directly to the page he or she originally tried to access. Direct Online Marketing™ typically does not employ this type of advertisement as part of its internet marketing services.

JavaScript – JavaScript – not to be confused with its distant cousin Java – is an Object Oriented Programming language developed by NetScape. It is used primarily to improve user experiences on websites with enhanced functionality.

Keyword – Almost interchangeable with Search Term, keywords are words or a group of words that a person may search for in a Search Engine. Keywords also refer to the terms you bid on through search engine marketing in trying to attract visitors to your website or Landing Page. Part of successful

Search Engine Optimization is including keywords in your website copy and Meta Tags.

Keyword Stuffing – When the Web was young and search engines were starting to gain in popularity, some smart website owners realized that the search engine Algorithms really liked some Meta Tags. Really liked them. So they started stuffing a bunch of keywords, often with high search volumes and no relevancy to the site, into title, description, and keyword tags. Sites instantly rocketed to great SERPs. Soon thereafter the search engines changed their ranking formulae and the sites lost their positions or were outright Banned.

Key Performance Indicator (KPI) – a particularly important performance measurement. A business may use KPIs to evaluate its success, or to evaluate the success of a particular activity in which it is engaged.

Keyword Tags – HTML tags which define the keywords used on Web pages. Meta keyword tags used to carry great weight with some older search engines until they caught up with the spammers using this practice and modified their algorithms. Today Google is officially on record for not giving these tags any weight.

Landing Page – The first page a person sees when coming to your website from an advertisement. This page can be any page on your website including your home page. Almost anytime you direct someone to your website from an advertisement, you should send them to a specialized landing page with tailored information to increase your landing page conversion rate. Radio advertisements are a notable exception as spelling out specific URL's can be time consuming and difficult to remember. Direct Online Marketing™ has extensive experience in creating, testing, and modifying landing page conversion rates to give your business the highest quality, least expensive, most cost effective leads possible.

Link Building – The process of obtaining hyperlinks (links) from websites back to yours. Link building is a crucial part of Search Engine Optimization.

Link Popularity – How many websites link to yours, how popular those linking sites are, and how much their content relates to yours. Link popularity is an important part of Search Engine Optimization, which also values the sites that you link out to.

Local Search – A huge and growing portion of the search engine marketing industry. Local search allows users to find businesses and websites within a specific (*local*) geographic range. This includes local search features on search engines and online yellow page sites. Optimizing for local search requires different practices than for traditional Search Engine Optimization.

Local Business Listings – Each of the major search engines offer local business listings that appear next to maps at the top of the page on many locally targeted searches. Business may either submit new requests or claim existing local business listings if the search engines have already added the company to the results. Having a website is not required for having a local business listing.

Long Tail Keywords – Rather than targeting the most common keywords in your industry, you can focus on more niche terms that are usually longer phrases but are also easier and quicker to rank for in the search engines. Long tail keywords can amount for up to 60% or so of a site's search traffic.

Meta Search Engine – A search engine that gets listings from two or more other search engines rather than crawling the Web itself.

Meta Tags (*see also keyword tags, description tags etc.*) – Meta tags allow you to highlight important Keywords related to your site in a way that matters to Search Engines, but that your website visitors typically do not see. Meta tags have risen and fallen in terms of valuation by internet marketers and search engines alike (*see Keyword Stuffing*), but they still play an important role in Search Engine Optimization.

Examples of meta tags include Header Tags and Alt Tags.

Microblogging – Microblogging refers to platforms allowing you to post information in snippets of 140 characters at a time via phone or Web. Twitter quickly became the dominant global player to the point where its name is synonymous with microblogging. In China, however, there are other popular microblogging services, generically called weibo.

Mobile Marketing– As cell phone technology advances, advertisers can not reach their target audience virtually anywhere. While mobile marketing is really just an extension of online marketing, it provides businesses many new opportunities and challenges.

Natural Listings – Also referred to as "organic results", the non-advertised listings in Search Engines. Some search engines may charge a fee to be included in their natural listings, although most are free. How high or low your website is ranked depends on many factors, two of the most important being content relevance and Link Popularity.

Naver – Naver is Korea's largest search engine and Web property. They offer paid search programs, although their pay per click program for non-Korean marketers has primarily been offered through Yahoo! / Overture – Korea. Naver's closest Korean competitor is Daum.

Opt-in – This type of registration requires a person submitting information to specifically request he or she be contacted or added to a list. Opt-ins typically lower lead flow rates and raise Costs per Acquisition from internet marketing campaigns, but may produce higher percentages of interested leads.

Opt-out – Here people are automatically signed up to receive contact, but can opt out of receiving newsletters, calls, etc. at any time.

Organic Listings –See Natural Listings.

Outbound Links – Links on any Web page leading to another Web page, whether they are within the same site or another website.

PageRank – PageRank is a value that Google assigns for pages and websites that it indexes, based on all the factors in its algorithm. Google does release an external PageRank scoring pages from 1-10 that you can check for any website, but this external number is not the same as the internal PageRank Google uses to determine search engine results. All independent search engines have their own version of PageRank. Potentially interesting fact: PageRank was named for Google's Larry Page and it is calculated at the page level – pun fun!

Paid Inclusion – Advertising program where pages are guaranteed to be included in a search engine's index in exchange for payment, though no guarantee of ranking well is typically given. For example, Looksmart is a directory that lists pages and sites, not based on position but based on relevance. Marketers pay to be included in the directory, on a CPC basis or a per-URL fee basis, with no guarantee of specific placement.

Paid Listings – Listings that search engines sell to advertisers, usually through paid placement or paid inclusion programs. In contrast, organic (natural) listings are not sold.

Paid Placement – See Paid Search below.

Paid Search –Also referred to as Paid Placement, Pay Per Click, and sometimes Search Engine Marketing, paid search marketing allows advertisers to pay to be listed within the Search Engine Results Pages for specific keywords or phrases. Paid placement listings can be purchased from a portal or a search network. Search networks are often set up in an auction environment where keywords and phrases are often associated with a cost-per-click (*CPC*) fee. Google AdWords and Yahoo! Search Marketing are the largest networks, but Microsoft adCenter (*live.com*) and other sites also sell paid placement listings directly as well.

A good search engine marketing company offering Paid Search will select an exhaustive set of industry-related Search Terms, set up your accounts, write advertising copy, create Landing Pages, control your bidding (*how much you're willing to pay per Search Term click*) and budgeting, and test and refine your advertising for effectiveness.

Pay-for-Performance – Term popularized by search engines as a synonym for pay-per-click, stressing to advertisers that they are only paying for ads that 'perform' in terms of delivering traffic, as opposed to CPM-based ads, which cost money, even if they don't generate a click.

Pay per Click (PPC) – See Cost per Click (*CPC*), above. The most common type of search engine advertising cost structure is PPC search engine marketing. Google, Yahoo, MSN, and many more search engines all use PPC.

Permission Marketing – Along the lines of Opt-in registrations, permission marketing focuses on receiving the consent of users before being contacted or, in some cases, even seeing an advertisement. Permission marketing is centered around the concept that people are increasingly tuning out the barrage of advertisements they see each day. Its focal tenet is that a business will have a better chance of gaining a client when the client first gives permission to be sent an ad or contacted. Search engine marketing by its nature can be thought of as a type of permission marketing – showing advertisements to people already searching for that information – as long as the ad is relevant to what they are searching.

Pop-Under – An advertisement that opens in a new Web Browser window once you visit a particular page or take some other action. Considered less annoying than Pop-Up ads because the new window appears behind the existing one.

Pop-Up – An extremely abused type of online marketing advertisement, pop-ups open new windows on your screen that partially or wholly cover your current Web Browser window. Some search engines ban ads that create a certain number (*or even any*) pop-up ads. Direct Online Marketing™ does not include pop-ups or pop-unders as part of its internet marketing services.

Press Optimization – The optimizing of press releases for search engines. This process has many similarities to Search Engine Optimization, although it focuses much more on Keyword use in content creation in regards to how press releases are often picked up by Blogs and other forms of new media.

Query – Query is another term for "keyword" or "search term." Within Google AdWords, search query reports show the *actual* terms that searchers used to click on your ads, as opposed to the *advertised* keyword that is in your account. These two sets of words may or may not be the same.

Rank – How well a particular Web page or website is listed in the Search Engine's Results. For example, a Web page about apples may be listed in response to a query for "apples."

However, "rank" indicates where exactly it was listed – be it on the first page of results, the second page or perhaps the 200th page. Alternatively, it might also be said to be ranked first among all the results, or 12th, or 111th. Overall, saying a page is "listed" only means that it can be found within a search engine in response to a query, not that it necessarily ranks well for that query. Also known as *position*.

Real Simple Syndication (RSS) – An increasingly popular new technology that allows information to be easily shared on websites or given directly to users per their request.

Reciprocal Link – A link exchange between two sites. Both sites will display a link to the other site somewhere on their pages. This type of link is generally much less desirable than a one-way inbound link.

Remarketing – Remarketing is Google AdWords's term for retargeting.
Results Page – Also referred to as a Search Engine Results Page.

Retargeting – Think of retargeting like cyberstalking. Someone performs an action (*often a visit to your site*) and has a cookie placed on her or his browser. Then as they go visiting other sites around the Web, your ad appears in front of them, as a banner or other type of display ad, on whatever sites they visit – so long as that site accepts ads from the ad network you use for retargeting. Retargeting can be done through various ad networks and platforms.

Return on Investment (ROI) – The key statistic for many companies: are your advertisements generating profits, and how much profit given the money you have had to pay. Direct Online Marketing™ always has its eye on ROI for all partners...and you should, too!

Rich Media – Web advertisements or pages that are more animated and/or interactive than static Banners or pages.
Robot or Bot – See *Crawler*.

Robots.txt – A file used to keep Web pages from being indexed or to tell which pages you want a search engine to index.

Run of Site (ROS) – A contract specifying Run of Site means that a Banner or other type of online advertisement can appear on any page, and usually in any open placement, of a particular website.

Scraping – The process of copying content from one Web property and using it on another. In other words, stealing. Scraping technologies have evolved because of the needs for content and to stay ahead of legitimate content creators trying to protect what they've written. Some companies offer content monitoring to help protect against scraping.

Search Engines – Search engines are places people go to search for things on the internet, such as Yahoo!, Google, or bing. Most search engines provide websites two ways of appearing: *Natural* (*free*) and Paid. Natural Listings, also referred to as organic listings, appear based on the search engines' own formulae. You can't pay to have your site listed higher (*although some search engines require that you pay to be included in the Natural listings*), but you can perform Search Engine Optimization (*SEO*). Paid Listings usually appear above or to the side of Natural listings and are typically identifiable as advertisements. The most common cost for advertising on Paid listings through Paid Search is Pay per Click (*PPC*).

Search Engine Marketing – All forms of marketing involving search engines – chiefly Search Engine Optimization and Paid Search Marketing. Sometimes this term will also be used to refer to *Paid Search* exclusively.

Search Engine Optimization (SEO) – A fancy way of saying "making your site search engine friendly". Search engine optimization is typically difficult to do on your own, especially given the increasing complexity and differences among all the search engines. Two important factors that rank highly in all major search engines are Link Popularity (how many websites – and how highly ranked those sites are – link to you) and relevant content (*how pertinent information on your website or a particular Web page is to a search*).

Search Engine Reputation Management (SERM) – Think of Search Engine Reputation Management as online spin control. SERM allows a person or organization better positioning through strategy involving Search Engine Optimization, Paid Search Marketing, Press Optimization, Blogging, and Social Media. The most important part of SERM is starting early – *before* a crisis.

Search Engine Results Page – Search Engine Results Pages, or SERPs, are the Web pages displayed by any Search Engine for any given search. They display both Natural (*organic*) Listings and Pay-Per-Click ads. How high you are listed and where your ad is shown depends on Search Engine Optimization; and paid Search Engine Marketing respectively.

Search Retargeting – A specific type of Retargeting that allows an advertiser to show ads to searchers of given keywords *who have never visited the advertiser's site*.

Search Terms – A search term is a word or group of words that a person types into a Search Engine to find what they are looking for. Based upon what a company sells, a website should incorporate the most popular or most popular specific search terms into the copy as Keywords. Figuring out the appropriate search terms to put into a website and to advertise on is a huge part of a Search Engine Marketer's job.

SEM – Acronym for search engine marketing and may also be used to refer to a person or company that does Search Engine Marketing – either Paid Search, Search Engine Optimization, or both.

SEO – Acronym for Search Engine Optimization and may also be used to refer to a person or company that does search engine optimization.

Site Retargeting – The most common form of retargeting: displaying your ads to a visitor based on a visit to your site, or individual page of your site. These cookie-based can appear on any publisher throughout the ad network being used. Various targeting options exist, including only showing ads when a certain page has been visited (*such as a landing page*) and an action has not been completed (*e.g. a conversion*).

Social Commerce - Selling goods directly online *through* through social media channels. Just like "*electronic commerce*" was shortened to "ecommerce", social commerce is sometimes shortened to "*s-commerce*" or "*f-commerce,*" the latter short for "facebook commerce."

Social Media - A type of online media where information is uploaded primarily through user submission. Web surfers are no longer simply consumers of content, but active content publishers. Many different forms of social media exist including more established formats like Forum and Blogs, and newer formats like Wikis, podcasts, Social Networking, image and video sharing, and virtual reality.

Social Networking – A type of Social Media, Social networking websites allow users to interact and create or change content on the site. These sites, of which businesses are now using for marketing purposes, allow users to create their own websites / online spheres (*e.g. LinkedIn and facebook*), share photographs (*e.g. flickr*), microblog / text small bits of information to their personal community (*e.g. twitter*) or recommend information for others to find on the Internet (*e.g. del.icio.us and Digg*). The sites in this last grouping are also referred to as social bookmarking or social news sites. There are also a growing number of sites that are heavily dependent on mobile and geographic locations, such as foursquare.

Spam – Can refer to unwanted data sent via email or put on a website to game a search engine. You're probably aware of spam in the classic email sense and hopefully also aware of the strict standards and penalties associated with the CAN-SPAM Act. Spam to a search engine is Web content that the search engine deems to be detrimental to its efforts to deliver relevant, quality search results. Some search engines have written guidelines about what they consider to be spamming, but ultimately any activity a search engine deems harmful may be considered spam, whether or not there are published guidelines against. Examples of spam include the creation of nonsensical doorway pages designed to pleased search engine algorithms rather than human visitors, or heavy repetition of search terms within a page (*i.e., the search terms are used tens or hundreds of times in a row*). Spam derives its name from a popular *Monty Python* skit.

Spider – A noun and a verb, Search Engines have spiders crawl through all the linked pages of a website to gather information to include the site in their Natural Listings and also use to determine their ranking on various Search Terms.

Stickiness – How often people return to a website. Constant updates, news feeds, and exclusive content are all ways to make a site stickier.

Submission – The act of submitting a URL for inclusion into a search engine's index. Unless done through paid inclusion, submission generally does not guarantee listing. In addition, submission does not help with rank improvement on crawler-based search engines unless search engine optimization efforts have been undertaken. Submission can be done manually (*i.e., you can fill out an online form and submit*) or automated, where a software program or online service may process the forms behind the scenes.

Tags – Words or phrases used to describe and categorize individual blog posts, videos, and pictures. Correctly using tags organizes content for users and can help with visibility through SEO and social media optimization.

Targeting – Shaping internet marketing campaigns to attract certain specific groups of prospective clients. Examples of Targeting include women, gun owners, and Medicare recipients. Behavioral Targeting is a newer, specific type of focus for advertisers.

Text Ad – An online advertisement that contains only written copy. Paid listings found on the results pages of the main Search Engines are currently Text Ads, although this is starting to change. Soon you should expect to see video ads pop up here occasionally.

TLD – TLD stands for Top Level Domain. The TLD is determined by whatever comes at the end of a domain name at its root – meaning without any page names.

Tracking Code – Information typically included in the URL that allows an advertiser to track the effectiveness of various aspects of an advertisement. Commonly tracked items include Search Term and referring Search Engine. 4th Generation Communications™ relies heavily on tracking code because tracking results is the only way to determine how effective our internet marketing services are.

Twitter Retargeting – Serving ads to people who have visited your site (or performed some other action) as promoted tweets or promoted accounts while they are on twitter. These ads go across devices, so you can reach visitors on mobile as well as desktop. Twitter is currently offering this type of advertising in beta only through a few select ad network partners.

URL – Uniform Resource Locator. These are the letters and symbols that make up the address of specific Web pages.

Unique Value Proposition (UVP) – In essence, what it is that sets your product, service, or company apart from others and why potential clients should care enough to choose you.

Universal Search – The placement of multiple types of results within a general search so that a user receives images, videos, local search results, news articles, and more next to general Web pages. Also called *blended search*.

Usability – How easy it is for a user to navigate a website and find the information he or she is seeking.

Viral Marketing – A newer method of internet marketing that attempts to make advertisements so interesting that viewers will pass them along to others free of charge to the advertisers.

Web 2.0 – A trendy buzzword for the internet marketing services industry, but also a legitimate idea and movement: the internet as a platform. Wikis, MySpace, and user-edited search all operate under this premise.

Web Browser – The program you use to access the internet. Common browsers include Microsoft Internet Explorer (IE), Apple's Safari, and Mozilla Firefox.

Webinar – "*Web Seminar*". These virtual seminars allow people from anywhere in the world to attend via an internet connection. They offer tremendous opportunities for businesses to reach out to people over large geographic areas at low costs.

Web Metrics – See Analytics.

Weibo – Weibo refers to microblogging in the Chinese market. Unlike the rest of the world where twitter is the only major player at this point, China has two major competing weibo services: Sina Weibo (#1) and Tencent Weibo (#2). A key advantage of these weibo platforms over twitter is the amount of information individual Mandarin characters can convey. Therefore, a single weibo post (*tweet*) of 140 characters can convey as much information as two paragraphs in English and other languages.

White Hat SEO – Used to describe certain Search Engine Optimization (*SEO*) methods, being "white hat" means using only SEO techniques that are completely above board and accepted by the Search Engines. Doing the opposite (*Black Hat*) can lead to your website seeing its rankings drop drastically – or being banned altogether

– even if the search engine optimization tactics aren't currently banned by search engines.

Wiki – A user-written, -controlled, and – edited site. Anyone with web access can change information appearing on Wikis, which can be about broad or specific topics. Wikis are becoming increasingly popular websites as people search for quality and (*hopefully*) unbiased information.

WordPress – WordPress is an extremely popular Content Management System. Developed originally for blogs, WordPress offers a great degree of flexibility and functionality.

XML – Extensible Markup Language. Content developers use this language with a variety of forms of content, including text, audio, and visual in order to allow users to define their own elements and pull the data at their pace. XML has played a huge part in the transformation of the Web towards Web 2.0.

Yandex – Yandex is the fastest growing search engine in the world, serving primarily Russia and other countries formerly part of the Soviet Union. It has been experimenting with an English-based search engine, but its main operations are for its Cyrillic engine. They do also offer a Google AdWords-like paid search program.

Z-Index – Using the z-index property of CSS allows you to better control positioning of overlapping elements. This element is sometimes used for black hat SEO purposes.

www.ingramcontent.com/pod-product-compliance
Lightning Source LLC
Chambersburg PA
CBHW051714170526
45167CB00002B/650